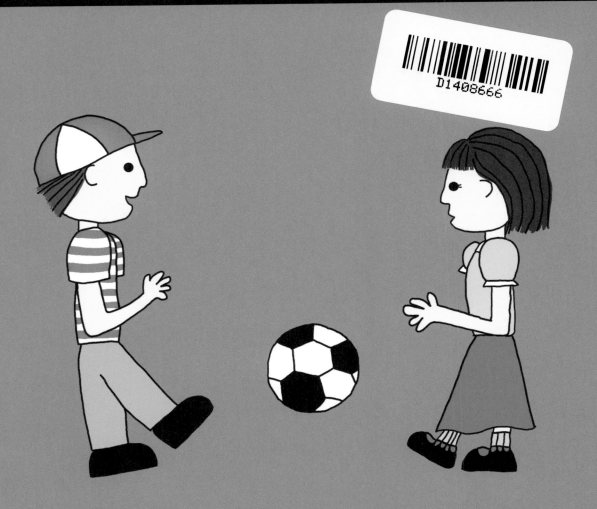

But most of the time I'm just a regular kid. I play like all the other kids.

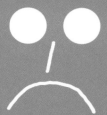

I get angry or sad just like my friends.

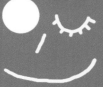

The Celiac Kid

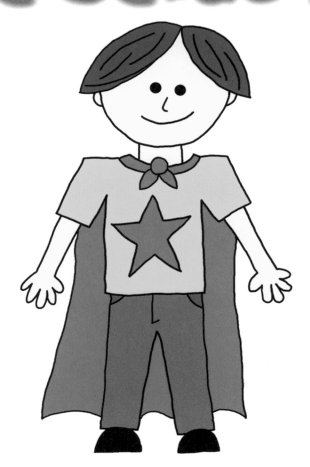

Written by Stephanie Skolmoski

Illustrated by Anneliese Bennion

ISBN 0-9786425-2-X

To Will, who will be a lifetime warrior against gluten and to a very supportive brother, Walker, who will fight by Will's side!

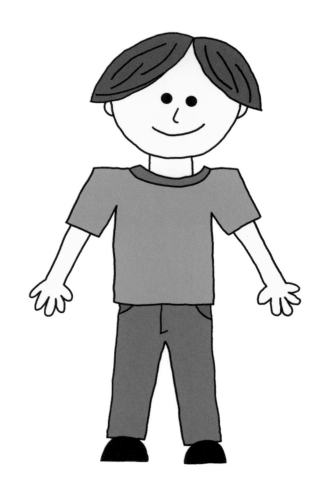

I am a celiac kid!

I'm okay with that. Sometimes it's hard.
Sometimes it's easy.

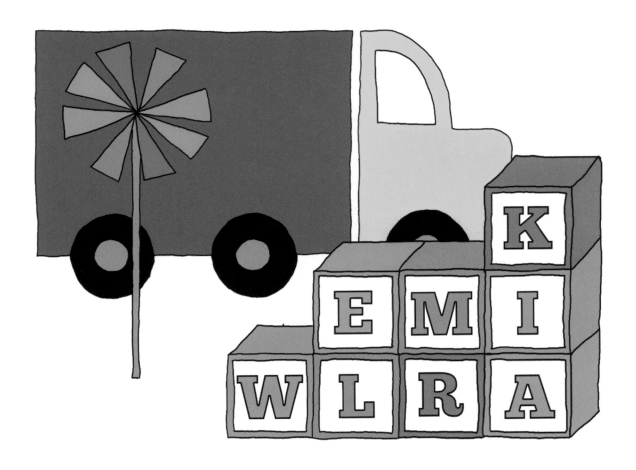

I love fans, cars and building stuff.

My mom and dad are the best on the planet.

My only archrival, as my dad puts it, is GLUTEN.

My body can't handle gluten. Gluten is in wheat, but it also hides in a lot of other food.

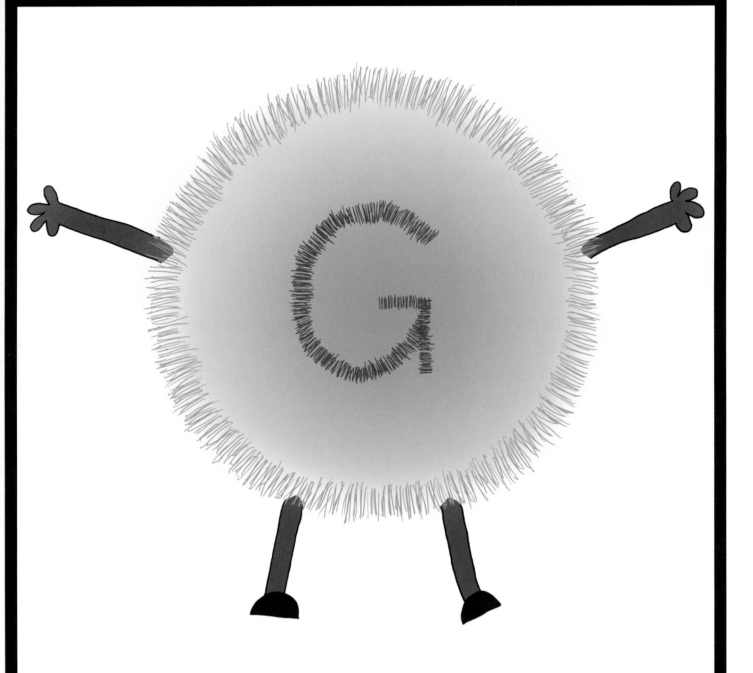

My parents and my grandparents are great readers of food labels because they love me.

Mom has found lots of sites on the Internet that really help.

You would be surprised where gluten hides. It can be in soy sauce, turkeys and even play dough! You've got be a good detective.

Nutrition Facts

Serving Size 50 g (1.8 oz)
Servings per Container 6

Amount per Serving

Calories 60   Calories from Fat 20

% Daily Value*

3%

6%

Total Fat 2g

Saturated Fat 1g

Trans Fat 0g

Polyunsaturated Fat 0g

Monounsaturated Fat 0.7g

Cholesterol 15mg

Sodium 15mg   Carbohydrate 7g

Fiber 1g

You might think that it's tough to be a celiac kid, but it's not so bad. I can eat fruits, veggies and all sorts of beans. In fact, most Mexican food is great.

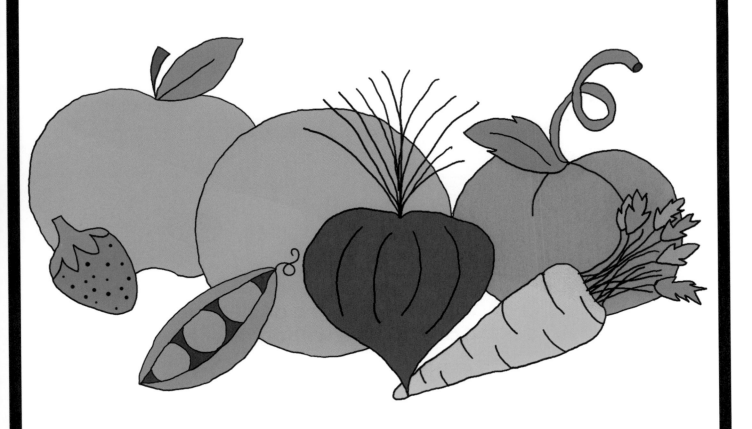

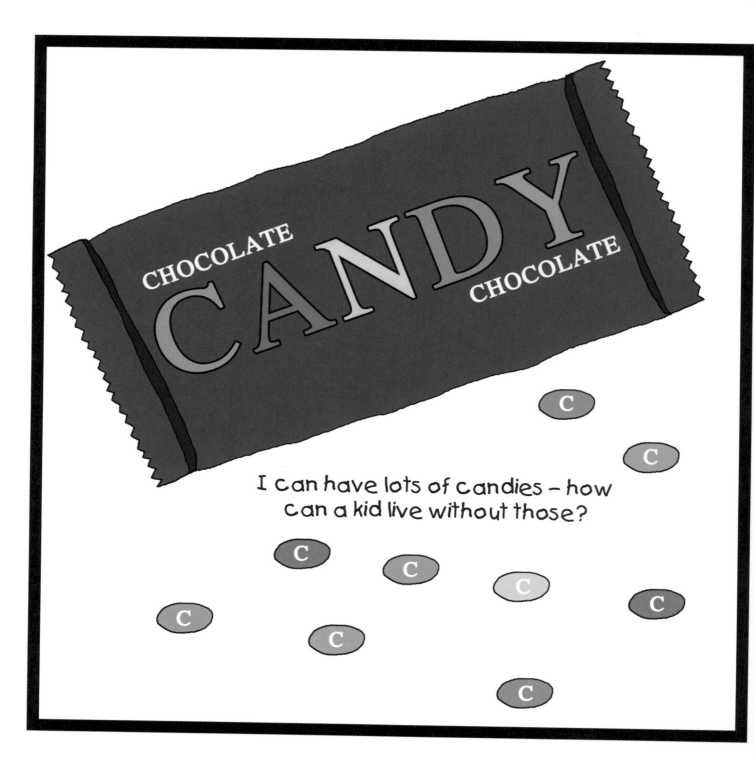

I can have lots of candies – how can a kid live without those?

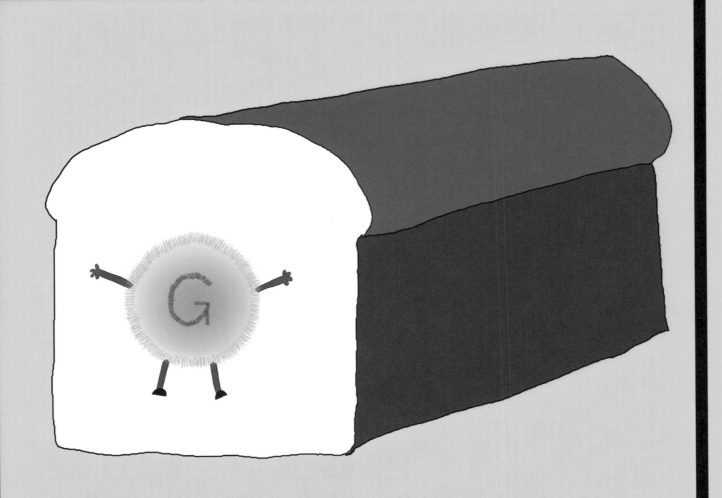

Probably the hardest thing to do without is bread. Mom and Dad take turns making bread for me each week with gluten-free flour.

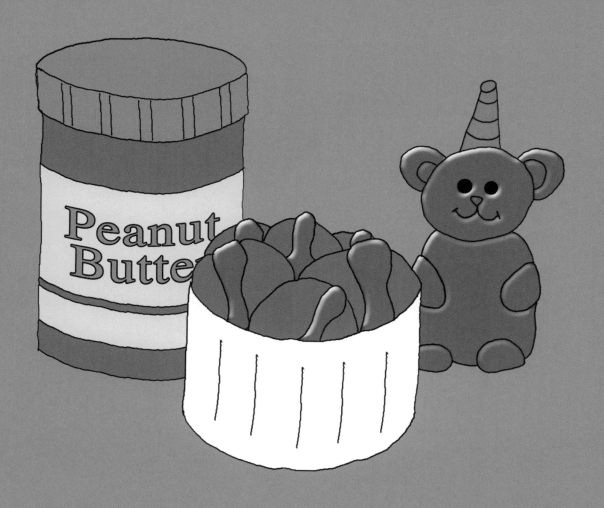

You see, I love PB and honey — A LOT.
Sometimes I just have a cup of peanut
butter with a squirt of honey. Oh, I love
that!

I love waffles and pancakes – gluten-free, of course. I especially like to dip them in syrup – what a treat! So you see, there are lots of different foods that I can eat.

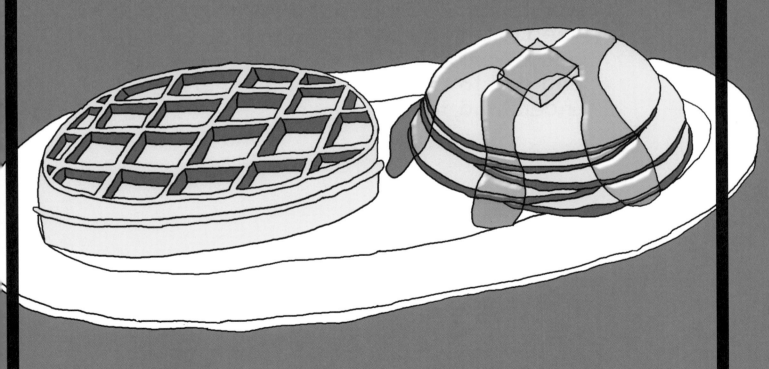

Let me tell you about celiac. My doctor is "Dr. Berry." Well that's what I call him. He is great and he is my "expert" celiac doctor.

Whenever I visit, he tells me things I need to know about celiac so I can be a super celiac kid. I can count on Mom and dad to listen so they can help me understand, too.

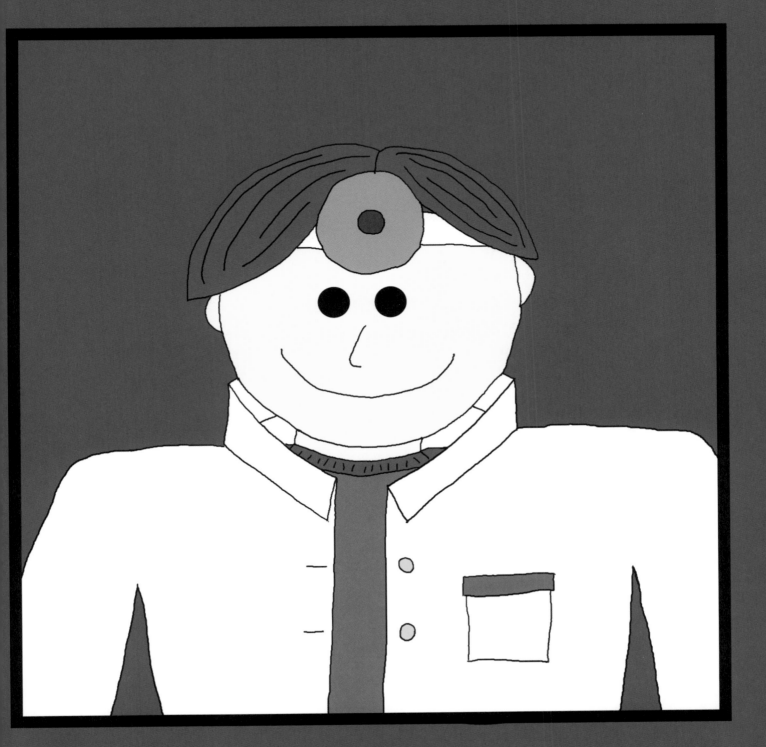

Here is what I know: Everyone has tiny villi in their intestines. They look like little pieces of hair.

Even though they are tiny, villi do wonderful work. They help our food go into our bodies so we can grow and our bodies can work the way they are supposed to.

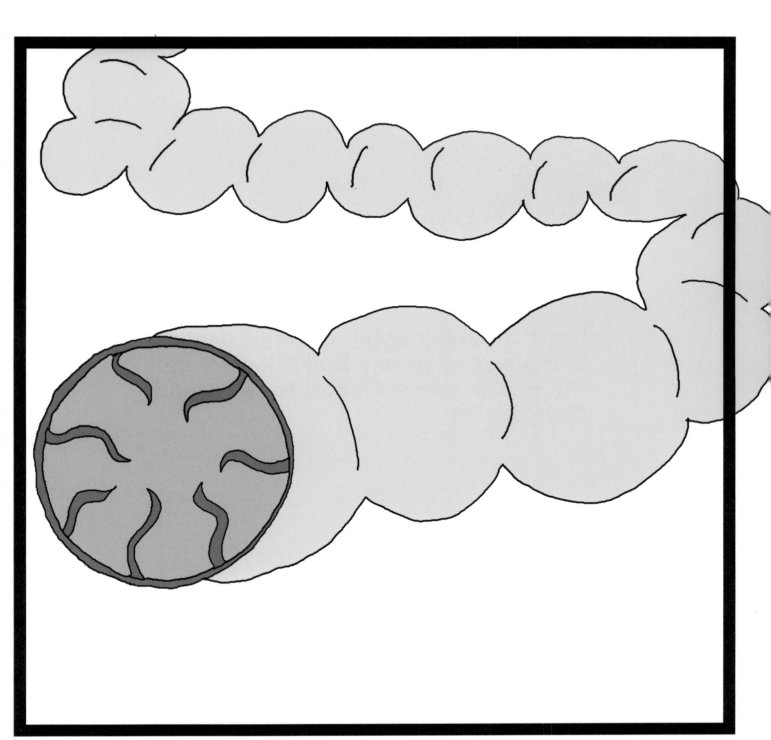

Because I have celiac disease, when I eat anything with gluten, the gluten destroys the little villi. Then my body can't use the food I eat.

I get a tummy ache, diarrhea (yuck!), and worst of all, my body doesn't get the nutrients that I need to grow and develop.

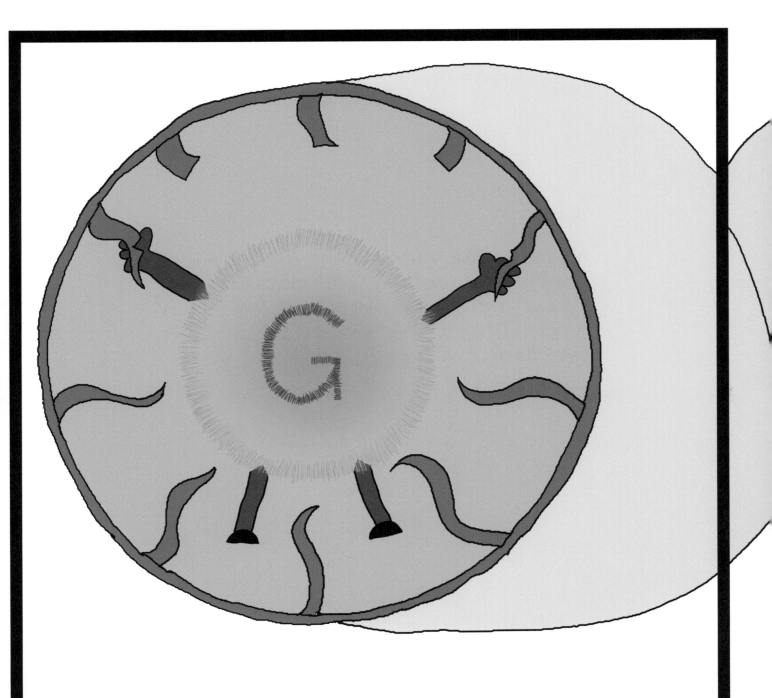

Nutrients are vitamins and minerals that our bodies need to work and grow. If I don't eat gluten, all my villi live. They help me digest my food so I can grow, feel good and be healthy.

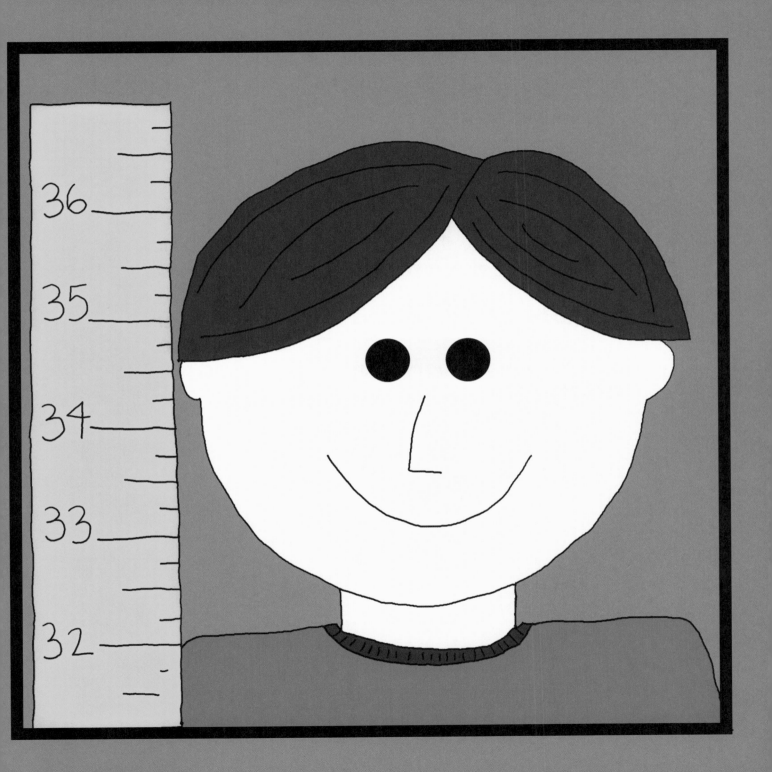

Now, mostly it's easy to be a celiac kid, but there are a few tough things about it.

I go to kindergarten – I love kindergarten, but when someone brings treats for their birthday, I usually can't eat any because there might be gluten in the treat.

Unfortunately, the whole world doesn't know that I am a celiac kid. Most people don't even know what that is!

So... my wonderful mom sends notes home to all the other moms telling them a little about me. In the note, she asks that when they bring treats for the class, to just let her know so she can send a treat just for me so I won't be left out.

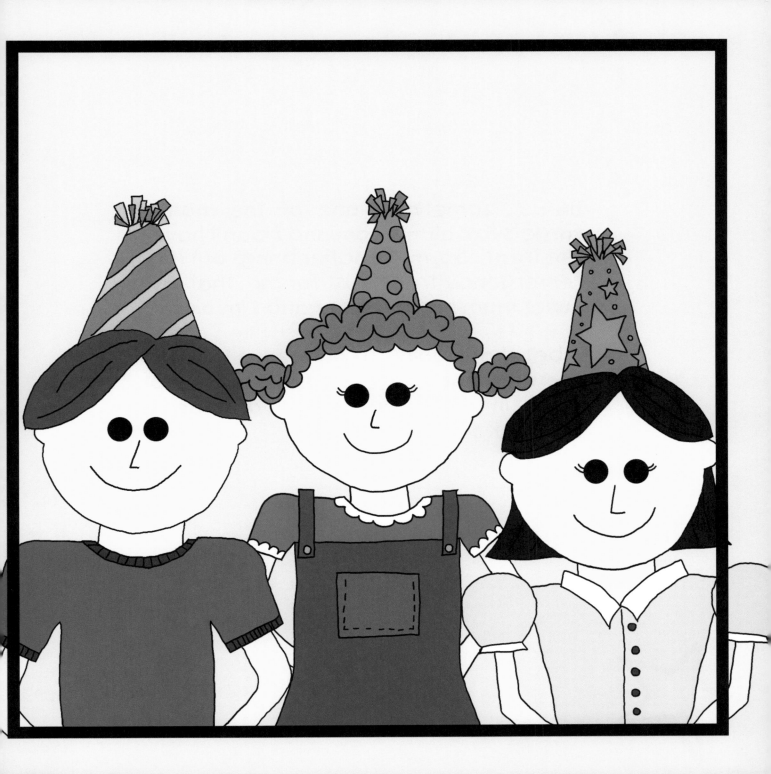

But. . . sometimes one of the moms forgets to call my mom and I can't have the treat. So, my teacher brings out the "emergency treat" just for me, that my super mom has given her and I'm okay.

I bet that's going to happen a lot as I grow up. But as I get bigger, I can keep treats in my locker or car. . . or even in my pocket!

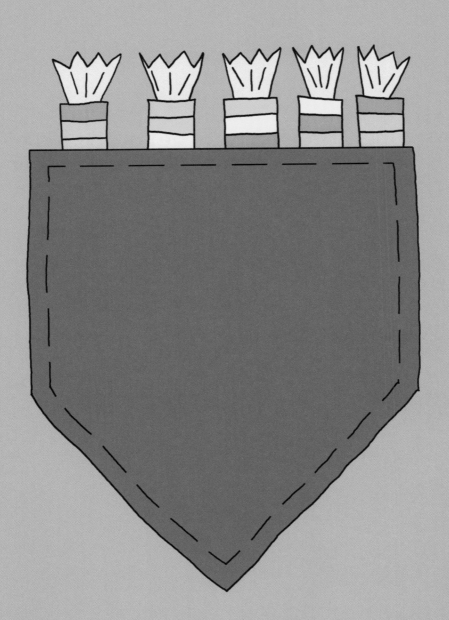

Another thing that can get a little tricky is when we get together with other people. Most of the time that means eating.

At picnics, I can have the hamburger or hot dog, but no bun. I can have corn on the cob and fruit. That's actually enough to fill me up.

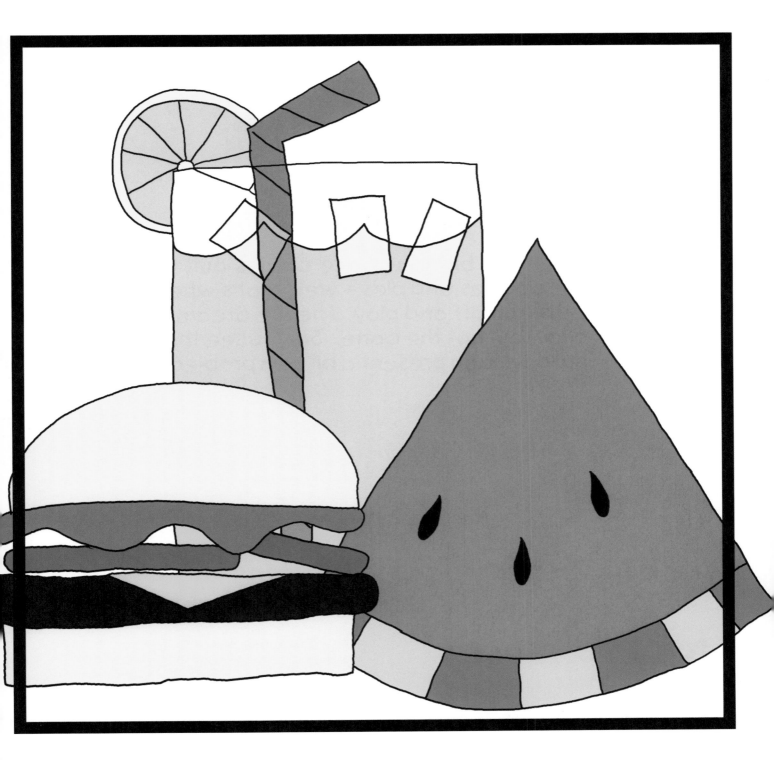

When the birthday cake comes out, or the cookies and pies – well, that's when I just run off and play. The ice cream is okay, but not the cone. So you see that holidays can present a bit of a problem.

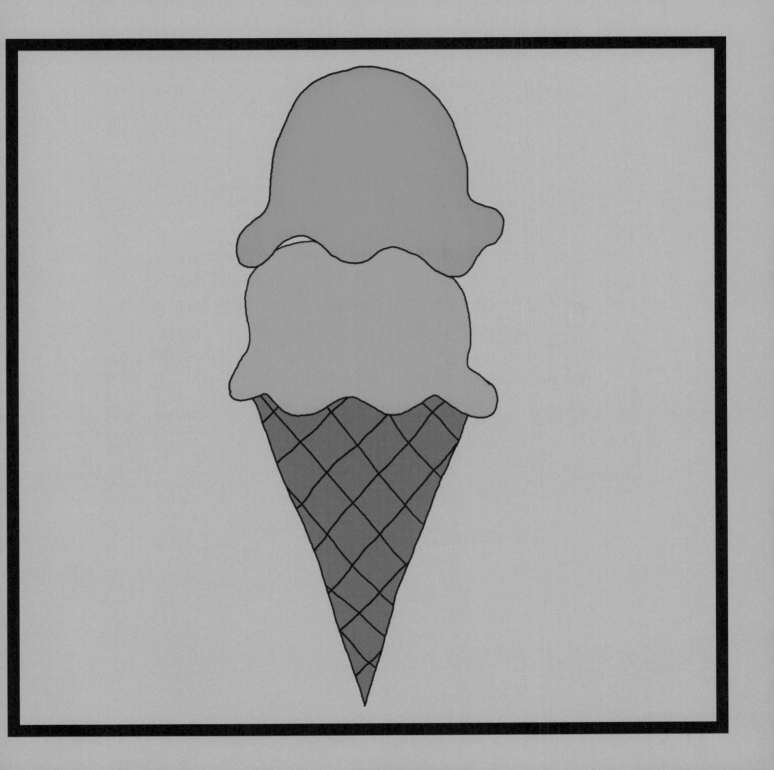

I am so glad that my mom lets people know as soon as we are invited to a party that I'm a celiac kid. We bring our own gluten-free food or we eat before we go. Then we just visit and play when we get together.

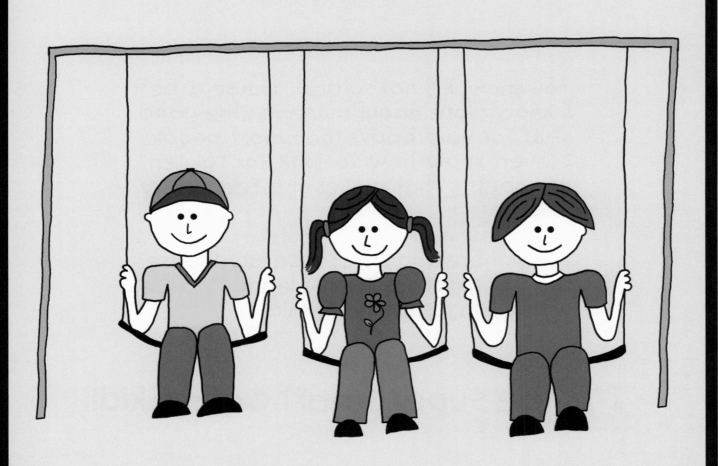

You know, it's not so bad, 'cause I bet I know more about nutrients (the good stuff for your body) than most people. I even know how to look for "gluten" on labels. That makes me feel pretty smart.

So far there is no cure for celiac disease, but I'm glad that I have learned to live with it. I'm just a smarter kid!

I'm the super smart celiac kid!

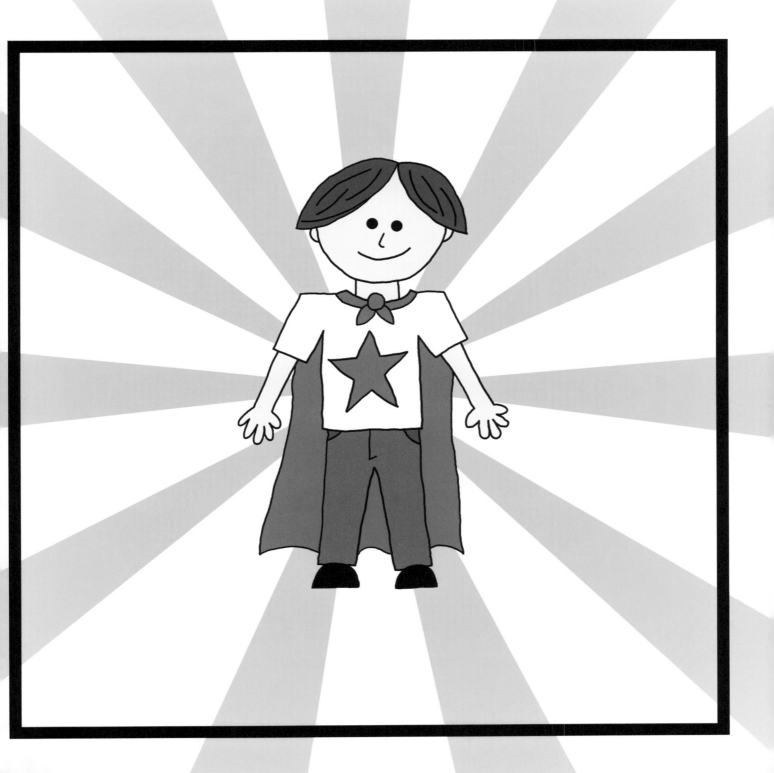

Stephanie Skolmoski loves to write – whether it's writing journals, short stories, poetry or children's musicals. In addition to raising five wonderful children, Stephanie has spent many years working with children and helping them love the arts. She has degrees in music and design.

Anneliese Bennion has doodled on paper since she could hold a pencil. She loves to create whimsical artwork and is fascinated with handwriting and fonts – she has even made up fonts of her own. She has a degree in design and works extensively in graphic design.

You can purchase more copies of this book at:

www.celiackidbook.com

See what else Stephanie & Anneliese have been up to at:

www.design-ability.com